Resistance Band Training

Learn to Use Resistance Bands to Maximize Your Workout and Improve Your Cardiovascular Health

By: NV Elite

Published in Canada

© Copyright 2015 – NV Elite

ISBN-13: 978-1518784378
ISBN-10: 1518784372

Table of Contents

Disclaimer 1

Introduction 3

Chapter 1: The Benefits of Strength and
Fucntional Training.. 5

    Strength Training Benefits.. 6

    Functional Training Benefits...................................... 7

    Flexibility and Mobility... 8

Chapter 2: The Reasons Why Resistance Bands
Work Better..11

    The Difference Between Resistance Bands and
    Free Weights.. 13

    Ability to Change Muscle Emphasis........................ 14

    Provides Linear Variable Resistance 14

Chapter 3: Resistance Loop Bands Outshine the
Rest...17

    Tube Bands... 18

    Therapy Bands 19

    Resistance Straps 19

    Loop Bands 20

Chapter 4: Resistance Bands are Convenient
and Cost Effective 23

    Resistance Bands are Easy to Mix and Match...... 25

Chapter 5: Effective Resistance Loop Band
Training Program 27

    Deadlifts Simulator... 28

    Squats.. 28

    Standing Glute Kick Backs 29

Kneeling Glute Kick Backs...29
Standing Leg Curls...30
Standing Side Leg Lifts 30
Push-ups..31
Seated Rows...31
Standing Biceps Curls 32
Standing Overhead Single Triceps Extension 32
Lying Down Leg Fly's 33
Glute Bridges 33
Standing Knee Lifts 34
Sitting Upright Rows 34
Reverse Fly's..35
Lower Body Training 38
Upper Body Training...39

Conclusion 41
Thank You! 41

Disclaimer

You should get your physician's approval before beginning any exercise program. These recommendations are not medical guidelines, but are for educational purposes only. You must consult your physician prior to starting any physical program or if you have any medical condition or injury that contraindicates physical activity. This program is designed for healthy individuals 18 years and older only.

The information in this report is meant to supplement, not replace, the proper exercise training. All forms of exercise pose some inherent risks. The editors and publishers advise readers to take full responsibility for their safety and know their limitations. Before practicing the exercises in this book, be sure that your equipment is well maintained, and do not take risks beyond your level of experience, aptitude, training and fitness. The exercise programs in this book are not intended as a substitute for any exercise routine or treatment or dietary regimen that may have been prescribed by your physician.

Don't lift heavy weights if you are alone, inexperienced, injured, or fatigued. Don't perform any exercise unless you have been shown the proper technique by a certified fitness trainer or certified strength and conditioning specialist. Always ask for instruction and assistance when lifting. Don't perform any exercise without proper instruction. Always do a warm-up prior to strength training and interval training. See your physician before starting any exercise program. If you are taking any medications, you must talk to your physician before starting any exercise program.

If you experience any lightheadedness, dizziness, or shortness of breath while exercising, stop the movement and consult a physician. You must have a complete physical examination if you are sedentary, if you have high cholesterol, high blood pressure, or diabetes, if you are overweight, or if you are over 30 years old. Please discuss all nutritional changes with your physician or a registered dietician.

Introduction

Many people believe that resistance band training is only a fad piece of equipment that will come and go, but resistance bands have been around for quite awhile and are now growing in popularity even more. The reasons why have to do with the ability to perform multiple types of training programs; the convenience of storage and transportation; and because they have actually been proven to work no matter how long they are used. You will come to find that there are many of other reasons why resistance bands are one of the cheapest and most effective pieces of equipment that you can own.

Trainers around the world are beginning to incorporate resistance bands into the daily workouts of their clients, and even elite athletes use them for a variety of different purposes on a weekly basis. Needless to say, the importance of resistance bands being utilized into daily workouts is quite high when it comes to keeping everything convenient and cost effective. Let's take a deeper look into the world of resistance band training, and see what benefits you will receive upon starting this type of workout.

4

Chapter 1:
The Benefits of Strength and Fucntional Training

Strength training and functional training go together like a pair of twins. They both provide a great deal of benefits for your body and are pretty easy to perform on a routine basis. The point of this chapter is to open your eyes to what the world of fitness has to offer our bodies, and the various types of equipment and techniques involved in making all this possible. In the end, all varieties of training are good for your body when properly performed, but the only difference is what best fits your schedule and costs.

Strength Training Benefits

Strength is not just for the massive bodybuilders, and is something that all of us need to function on a daily basis. Every step you take requires strength, and even being able to stand for a long period of time displays leg and lower back strength. So what exactly is this type of training? Strength training is when you use your muscles to contract against a resistance in the hopes of achieving greater strength and endurance in the muscle groups being targeted.

This kind of training is not just for strength. Your bone density begins to become stronger as well. Doctors are now recommending strength training utilization for men and women of all adult ages since this is what keeps your body's skeletal muscles functioning properly. Even people in their senior years are being advised to perform this at least 2-3 days a week, which helps prevent sudden fractures from occurring due to stronger bones. Frequent strength training performed correctly may also prevent arthritis and osteoporosis.

Resistance bands play a key role in this since they produce resistance that your muscles must contract to overcome, and they are being used quite often for this type of training now. People generally use them alone as the only form of resistance during the exercise, but recently more and more power lifters are beginning to realize that these bands have many beneficial uses.

On top of all these benefits, you also can look forward to an increase in your metabolism, which encourages fat loss.

Functional Training Benefits

Functional training is basically performing exercises that relate to real world applications. Almost all exercises you perform are going to assist you with your daily life outside of the gym, but this training is to specifically target certain movements that are more beneficial for either your body as a whole, or for certain areas such as your lower trunk. For example, if you have to walk up two flights of stairs routinely, then you would perform variations of lunges, which simulate the muscle movements used for walking up the stairs.

Strength training mixes well with this because usually you want some type of resistance to actually get a solid training session in. Without this you are performing Calisthenics, which is more used for flexibility and body maintenance opposed to muscle strengthening. Sure, performing pushups regularly builds body strength, but after performing them so often there is that dreaded feeling of performing them when you require doing a higher amount of repetitions.

Resistance bands come into the equation when you think about being able to use a device that is un-stable and easy to manipulate.

Dumbbells and barbells are in set forms and only have a few types of motions to perform with them since they are stable. Un-stable is being able to move the resistance in almost all different directions that you choose. Resistance bands and kettlebells fall into this category and are known for being the best equipment both at the gym and in the home.

Flexibility and Mobility

Without flexibility and mobility, we face a challenge performing even the simplest strength training exercises since injury may occur, or your muscles may even fatigue too early as well. Flexibility and mobility are basically being able to lift an object without injuring your back, or reaching for an object on the top shelf without pulling your shoulder muscles. Various forms of stretching increase these components of life, and resistance bands help increase the benefits of stretching further. While stretching, you are usually allowing gravity to pull the weight of your body into the stretch, or sometimes you have to manually cause the pull on your own.

Using a resistance band allows you to increase the tension placed on your muscles during the stretch, thus allowing them to fully warm up by hitting deep into the muscle tissues. Resistance loop bands are particularly great for this purpose – especially when it comes to your lower body muscles.

All of these different factors are involved when it comes to turning your body into great shape. Strength training allows the skeletal muscles to become stronger and less prone to injury, and is what allows functional training to be even greater than it already is. Do not be afraid to add weighted resistance into your training programs, and that is why resistance bands come quite handy.

Resistance bands are capable for being used in all variations of training described in this chapter, and in the next chapter you will see why they are possibly more beneficial than other types of equipment. This is not to say that exercising with free weights and other variations of strength training equipment is a bad thing, but there are certain advantages that only resistance bands are capable of bringing to the table.

"No citizen has a right to be an amateur in the matter of physical training...what a disgrace it is for a man to grow old without ever seeing the beauty and strength of which his body is capable." - Socrates

Chapter 2:
The Reasons Why Resistance Bands Work Better

People often look at resistance bands in a bad way since they appear to do little for the body. The reason for this is because they are small, string-like, and weigh very little. We are often taught that the more weight being used is better for training, but nobody really reinforces the fact that everything depends on resistance – not volume. Resistance bands do share similar qualities to free weights by providing benefits such as:

Free range of motion
Some type of muscle strengthening resistance
Progressive resistance
Variable speeds of movement

What this list tells you is that resistance bands and free weights both provide resistance that you can adjust the speed and weight of the resistance being created. Studies show that these bands are capable of providing the same strength, fat loss, and muscle gaining benefits as free weights do.

The reason for this is because our bodies have no idea what we are using to create the resistance placed against our muscles for contraction. For example, you have a dumbbell, kettlebell, resistance band, and tree branch that all provide the same amount of weighted resistance. If you took all these items and performed biceps curls, your body would not be able to distinguish any difference between them, and muscle hypertrophy will occur regardless of the equipment used. For this reason, the myth that only heavy free weights increase muscle growth is just that – a myth.

The Difference Between Resistance Bands and Free Weights

They both provide strength training benefits and can be used for functional training, but there are some qualities found in resistance bands only. These qualities would be:

Gravity is not a factor
Ability to change muscle emphasis
Provides linear variable resistance

Let's touch base on how gravity affects your workout with equipment. Free weights are cumbersome devices that require gravity to create resistance. The movements are stuck to a vertical plane, which means you can only create resistance with a free weight by moving it up or down. For example, if you took a dumbbell and pressed it over your head, the resistance is being created. However, if you move the dumbbell from the left side of your body to the right, you notice there are no muscles under tension aside from the ones being used to grasp the dumbbell.

Resistance bands require no gravity to create muscle contraction. You will always feel tension no matter which way you stretch the resistance band.

This is the reason why even athletes are constantly using resistance bands since they can cause muscle contractions on functional areas that dumbbells are not able to do since gravity is not a factor. Exercises performed on a horizontal plane allow better functional training to prevent injuries from performing daily actions such as turning with a box.

Ability to Change Muscle Emphasis

The ability to change muscle emphasis is being able to keep resistance on a specific muscle group. Let's take a look at biceps curls for a better example. When using dumbbells, you create resistance against your biceps on the vertical plane, but once the dumbbell passes your bicep muscle the gravity just drags it back, which makes the resistance fade away. Elastic bands and tubes are different because resistance is being generated the entire time due to gravity not having any effects on the exercise.

Provides Linear Variable Resistance

This is one of the most important differences between elastic resistance and free weight resistance. While using a free weight, you only have that set amount of resistance to place against your muscles, so whatever muscle fibers are being used is it. However, elastic resistance is always increasing throughout the exercise movement. When you perform an exercise, the band starts off with little to no tension.

While the range of motion begins to increase, so does the resistance due to the fact that they are elastic, and as it gets pulled more tension begins to form. Then during the second phase of the exercise, the resistance is still there since gravity is not allowing you to simply lower the weight quickly.

Chapter 3:
Resistance Loop Bands
Outshine the Rest

Okay, you now have a better understanding of resistance bands and their many uses, but let's take a look at the different types of resistance bands available to you. The primary types are tube bands, therapy bands, and loop bands, which all have their own separate varieties within each category. Each variation will have different uses for it, but generally you can use any kind of resistance band to perform most exercises. Let's take a look at these elastic bands to get a better feel for what is available.

Tube Bands

This is the more common type of resistance bands that you will encounter. They are made of elastic materials shaped into a tube. They usually have two foam handles attached to make it easier for gripping and holding in the palms of your hands. The resistance takes a little longer to set in for more than half the exercises when it comes to regular sizing, but some brands are shorter for this reason.

Resistance tube bands are generally color coded from lightest color being the lightest resistance, and darker colors being the strongest. Everything depends on the brand, so make sure to review their resistance chart before making a purchase.

You can find these with an assortment of features such as being multilayered with the rubber, which is what makes them stronger, durable, and in the end last longer than single layer rubber tubes. Another type of outer layering is a cloth-like protector sometimes found as braided for extra reinforcement. These features make them cost almost as much as a dumbbell though.

Therapy Bands

Resistance straps were used for several decades as tools to help rehabilitate the injured, so therapy bands get their name for this reason. They are generally lighter in resistance, and share the same similarities as loop bands by being flat and circular in shape. Use these for lighter tasks such as exercises being performed for shoulder recovery. People do use these therapy bands for training, but mainly as a means for stretching opposed to strength training.

Resistance Straps

Here is another type of resistance band that needs to be covered. Resistance straps are usually flat and have a little extra length to them. They are designed to be used as either a strap, or you can tie the ends together to make a loop band. People even tie one end to a stable device and perform exercises with the other end. Resistance straps are versatile and can be used for a lot of different methods, but the straps tend to be a little thinner with most brands, which means they can possibly tear under too much resistance.

Loop Bands

Loop bands are becoming one of the best elastic bands available for a cheap price since they a durable and provide a lot of resistance since they cannot be stretched too far. They are generally said to be for core and lower body exercises, but there are a variety of loop band exercises that focus on muscle groups all around your body. Their overall design is pretty basic since it is a flat band fully developed into a circle. They come in a variety of sizes, but normally the smaller ones are used for high resistance desires.

One of the best things about loop bands is the fact that they are completely ready to use in a circle, which allows you to place it under your feet, or around your thighs and ankles. The compact design keeps resistance in place for most exercises before you even begin the motions. For example, when you place a loop band around your lower thigh area, you have to place your feet at least shoulder width apart.

This causes the band to stretch and provide immediate resistance, and as you drop your hips for the squat, your thighs push out following your knees, which then causes greater and increasing resistance throughout the squats you are performing.

Loop bands are also unique to the rest because they can be used for isometric training and still provide resistance. Isometrics are when you perform an exercise that does not require any body movement that causes a joint to move, which means you are stable and still. A good example of this would be the planks. The resistance loop band adds extra training capabilities since, as mentioned before, the resistance is already being placed as you're getting into position. Use this technique for isometric exercises such as planks, wall sits, and pushups (maintain the mid pushup position).

Chapter 4:
Resistance Bands are
Convenient and Cost Effective

This chapter discusses advantages of resistance training from a non-physical perspective. People spend hundreds, if not thousands, of dollars on multiple fitness machines to own in their own home, and this includes dumbbells, barbells, benches, and the weight plates to go with them. All of this equipment is almost unthinkable to fit inside your home, and is not even of any use if you have to travel and take care of other affairs that keep you away from home. Why own all of this when you can purchase a few resistance bands for pennies compared to the other types of equipment?

Resistance bands are a cost effective approach to having equipment that provides strength training benefits with little money out of pocket needed. You can walk into most merchandise stores and find a resistance band ready to be used, and a lot of times they tend to go on sale as well. Remember, these elastic bands are capable of performing more tasks for your muscles than the average free weights, and free weights generally get priced per pound/kilogram. That ends up costing a lot more than a resistance band that provides the same results.

Then there is the convenience of sticking to training programs focusing on resistance bands. They are easy to move around since bands generally weigh a lot less than a pound, and then they are able to be folded or wrapped up to carry inside of a backpack or suitcase. You can travel for vacation and bring your resistance training with you with little effort. Training in the convenience of your own home is also a perk that comes along with resistance band training. You can easily keep yourself safe and out of any bad weather while owning these, and there is no fee or contract from needing to attend a gym for their equipment.

Resistance Bands are Easy to Mix and Match

Yes, the best benefit is being able to do everything with resistance bands only, but what about adding them into your already set strength training programs? These bands can be used to mix with your other exercises that use things such as free weights. For example, the resistance band is great for burnouts. Perform a set of barbell curls, and then immediately follow them with resistance band curls. You will feel your muscles burn to the multiple forms of resistance. Next, you can add them into compound lifts since they add extra resistance to the movement. There really is no reason why you cannot mix all types of equipment to get a functional workout in.

Chapter 5:
Effective Resistance Loop Band Training Program

First, you will be given the exercises that will be used for this program, and then a description of what they are used for and how to perform them. Usually you can perform the exercises interchangeably with your workouts, but beginners should stick to the program for at least 4 weeks before embarking on making any changes. Once you reach the point to where you feel more exercises need to be added, begin to find new ones that involve the same muscle groups and change them out every few weeks.

Deadlifts Simulator

The deadlift is one of the most effective compound lifts that target muscles in almost your entire body. Primary areas include all leg muscles, lower back, and hip flexors. We say this is a simulator since the barbell is used mainly for this exercise. Step: [1] Place loop band underneath feet and spread legs shoulder width apart. [2] Bend at your hips to grasp free section of loop band. [3] Keeping your back straight and chest out pull your upper body back up while holding onto the loop band. [4] Straighten body out and repeat until complete.

Squats

A squat is equally as important to perform as the deadlift is. Primary muscle groups being focused on are your glutes, quads, and hamstrings, although most of your leg muscles get a good workout as well. Step: [1] Step inside loop band and slide it up until it is approximately 2 inches above your knees. [2] Position feet shoulder width apart and hold hands out in front of you. [3] Keeping your back straight and chest out, begin to drop your hips back and squat down until you are low enough to sit in a chair. [4] Drive your hips forward and stand back up in starting position for next repetition.

Standing Glute Kick Backs

This exercise is great for targeting your glutes, hamstrings, and hip flexors. This is one of the easiest exercises to perform, but also one of the most beneficial. Step: [1] Step inside the loop and slide it to just above your ankles. [2] With a foot gap between your feet, slightly lean forward and push back one foot with legs fully extended. [3] Bring your foot back to resting position and repeat. Exercise is to be alternated to matching sets per leg.

Kneeling Glute Kick Backs

The kneeling version of the kickback is able to get a little more muscle contraction to your glutes while using a loop band. Primary muscles being targeted are your glutes, hamstrings, and thighs. Step: [1] Kneel on all fours and slide the loop band just below both knees. [2] Place your palms on the ground and have your knees pointing forward. [3] Push one leg back as you push it outwards as well to keep tension on the band. [4] Push far enough back until you feel your glutes tighten firmly. [5] Lower your knee back to the ground and repeat exercise. Next, alternate to your other leg after set is complete.

Standing Leg Curls

Leg curls are great for your hamstrings, and the standing version also helps out with your balance and flexibility as well. Step: [1] Stand inside of loop band and slide it to just below your calf. [2] Keeping your knee in place, begin to pull one foot directly up and towards your glutes. [3] Stop the movement once your heel has passed the back of your knees. [4] Lower your foot back down and repeat. Ensure you alternate between legs after each set is complete.

Standing Side Leg Lifts

The movement for this exercise is not only great for strength training, but also helps with balance as well. Muscle groups targeted are your hips, thighs, and abdominal muscles primarily. A light resistance may be required at first since it is a more difficult exercise to perform. Step: [1] Step inside loop and slide it up above your ankles. [2] Spread feet apart just enough to cause the band to stay in place above ankles. [3] Keeping your leg straight begin to push and raise one foot directly to the side of your body while leaning your upper body the opposite direction. [4] Lower foot back down and repeat. Exercise is to be alternated to matching sets per leg.

Push-ups

The number one upper body strengthening exercise has just gotten better with the loop band. Muscles targeted are your chest, shoulders, and triceps primarily. Step: [1] Lie down on the ground stomach down and body fully extended. [2] Slide loop band over your head and place it beneath your armpits. [3] Place the palms of your hands on the free side of your loop band. [4] Perform the push-up as you normally would and feel the burn!

Seated Rows

This exercise is another "must-do" for targeting muscles in your upper body. Primary muscles being used are your upper back, shoulders, and biceps. Step: [1] Sit on the floor and extend your legs fully out, feet together, with heels on the floor. [2] Take the elastic band and place it down the center of each foot. [3] Lean forward and grasp the loop band with palms facing down. [4] Keeping your back straight slightly lean back and pull the band to your mid section. Allow the band to reset and repeat the exercise movements.

Standing Biceps Curls

The biceps curl is one of the most common exercises you will see performed, and they allow you to build your arm strength. Primary muscles targeted are your biceps and forearms. Step: [1] Place loop band underneath your right foot. [2] Grasp the other portion of the band with your right hand and stand straight up again. [3] With your elbow in and arm fully extended down, begin to curl the weight up to your right shoulder. Make sure you are not leaning back to complete the movement. [4] Allow the band to retract and repeat the exercise steps. Alternate to left side after set is complete.

Standing Overhead Single Triceps Extension

Your triceps are the largest arm muscle and need a good workout in order to keep your arms growing equally. The primary muscle being targeted is your triceps, but your forearms and shoulder joints get a nice workout as well. Step: [1] Grasp the end of the loop in your left hand, and then place it against your lower back. [2] Ensuring you do not overstretch your shoulder, grasp the other end of the loop with your right hand. [3] Pull the band up above your head and out to the right side of your body. Complete the set and alternate to next arm.

Lying Down Leg Fly's

Your inner thighs and hips are going to love this exercise, but the only difference from the machine is that you only move one leg each set. Step: [1] Lie on your side and place your legs inside the loop. [2] Slide the loop band up until just above your knees and then place a slight bend in them. [3] Using the leg that is NOT against the floor, begin to open your legs apart until you reach maximum movement. Repeat and then alternate the side you lay on.

Glute Bridges

Glute bridges primarily target your glutes of course, but they also help strengthen your hips, lower back, and abdominal muscles, which are basically the core of your body. Step: [1] Lie on your back and slide the loop band approximately 2 inches above your knees. [2] Place your feet together and slide them in towards your buttocks until your legs are open - similar to a squat. [3] Keeping your shoulders and feet against the floor, slowly begin to drive your hips forward until you have a slight tension in your lower back. Slowly repeat this movement.

Standing Knee Lifts

This exercise creates a different type of workout when performed with a resistance loop band. Muscles targeted are your glutes, quads, and hip flexors as well. Step: [1] Place the band underneath your right foot, and then slide the other half over the top of your left foot. [2] Stand with your feet hip-width apart, upper body straight, and place your hands on your hips for support. [3] Simply raise your left knee up until your upper leg is parallel with the floor. Repeat the exercise and then alternate to right leg training.

Sitting Upright Rows

Upright rows place your shoulder joints under a lot of contraction and feel great to perform. The primary muscle groups targeted are your shoulders and traps. Step: [1] Take a seat and fully extend your legs out with feet together. [2] Place the loop band around the center of each foot, and then grasp the band with both hands facing palms down. [2] Slightly lean your upper body back and pull the band to your chin. Your elbows should flare up towards your ears.

Reverse Fly's

This exercise places a lot of emphasis on your upper back muscles along with your shoulders as well. The movement may take a few tries to get down, but an overall effective exercise to perform. Step: [1] Standing or sitting, place your body inside the loop band and position it just below your armpits. [2] Pull your elbows in and slide your forearms into the other side of the loop until it is halfway down your forearms. [3] Push your arms out and away from your body until you feel your upper back muscles squeeze and contract.

Now, let's place all of these exercises together into a resistance loop band training program you can perform up to 4 days a week. You want at least 24 hours between each training day for muscle recovery and repair, but 48 hours of rest is recommended for people new to fitness training.

Squats: **x2 sets for x12-15 repetitions**

Deadlift Simulator: **x2 sets for x12-15 repetitions**

Seated Rows: **x2 sets for x12-15 repetitions**

Kneeling Glute Kick Backs: **x2 sets for x12-15 repetitions**

Pushups: **x2 sets for x12-15 repetitions**

Standing Leg Curls: **x2 sets for x12-15 repetitions**

Standing Biceps Curls: **x2 sets for x12-15 repetitions**

Standing Side Leg Lifts: **x2 sets for x12-15 repetitions**

Standing Glute Kick Backs: **x2 sets for x12-15 repetitions**

Squats: **x2 sets for x12-15 repetitions**

Congratulations, you have completed your first resistance loop band exercise. Your body will most likely begin to feel sore and achy by the next morning, so make sure you eat plenty of nutrients and stretch your muscles to keep the soreness away. After you feel this is not enough for your body's workout, you should add an extra set to each exercise given. Repeat up to x5 sets each before changing any exercises in and out of the program.

However, you may prefer to train your lower and upper body muscles separately, and this is okay since many people prefer this method to train with. Let's start with lower body training and then alternate with upper body training.

The weekly fitness program differs since you will be training back-to-back for 4 days, and then rest for three. You can do this since your training schedule is - lower, upper, lower, upper, and then day 5 is open.

You have the option to add in an abdominal specific training program of your choice on day 5 of the week if you wish, or a third day of lower body training. If you wish to have a third day of upper body training, you need to start the week with the upper body workout. Remember to add another set with each exercise after you get used to the movements.

Lower Body Training

Squats: x2 sets for x12-15 repetitions
Standing Knee Lifts: x2 sets for x12-15 repetitions
Standing Side Leg Lifts: x2 sets for x12-15 repetitions
Standing Glute Kickbacks: x2 sets for x12-15 repetitions
Standing Leg Curls: x2 sets for x12-15 repetitions
Lying Down Leg Fly's: x2 sets for x12-15 repetitions
Glute Bridges: x2 sets for x12-15 repetitions
Kneeling Glute Kick Backs: x2 sets for x12-15 repetitions
Squats :   x1 set until muscle failure

Upper Body Training

Deadlift Simulator:	**x2 sets for x12-15 repetitions**
Seated Rows:	**x2 sets for x12-15 repetitions**
Sitting Upright Rows:	**x2 sets for x12-15 repetitions**
Push-Ups:	**x2 sets for x12-15 repetitions**
Reverse Fly's:	**x2 sets for x12-15 repetitions**
Standing Biceps Curls :	**x2 sets for x12-15 repetitions**
Standing Overhead Triceps Extensions:	**x2 sets for x12-15 repetitions**
Seated Rows:	**x1 set until muscle failure**

Conclusion

You now have a great understanding of how resistance bands are beneficial for people of all different ages and genders. The exercises provided have been designed to target every muscle group at least once during the training day. Always make a habit to stretch your muscles and joints prior to training, which is going to help prevent any muscle strains from occurring since your body is warmed up. Remember, you are advised to seek consultation with a physician before embarking on a new fitness program if you have had any medical conditions in the past. Stay safe and train properly.

Thank You!

DISCLAIMER AND/OR LEGAL NOTICES: Every effort has been made to accurately represent this book and it's potential. Results vary with every individual, and your results may or may not be different from those depicted. No promises, guarantees or warranties, whether stated or implied, have been made that you will produce any specific result from this book. Your efforts are individual and unique, and may vary from those shown. Your success depends on your efforts, background and motivation.

The material in this publication is provided for educational and informational purposes only and is not intended as medical advice. The information contained in this book should not be used to diagnose or treat any illness, metabolic disorder, disease or health problem. Always consult your physician or health care provider before beginning any nutrition or exercise program. Use of the programs, advice, and information contained in this book is at the sole choice and risk of the reader.